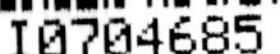

VitAMIN
D
Antioxidants
HEART HEALTHY
COOKBOOK
For Beginners
SIMPLE GUIDE TO COOKING WITH LOVE
FOR YOUR HEART
MARGARET M GORE

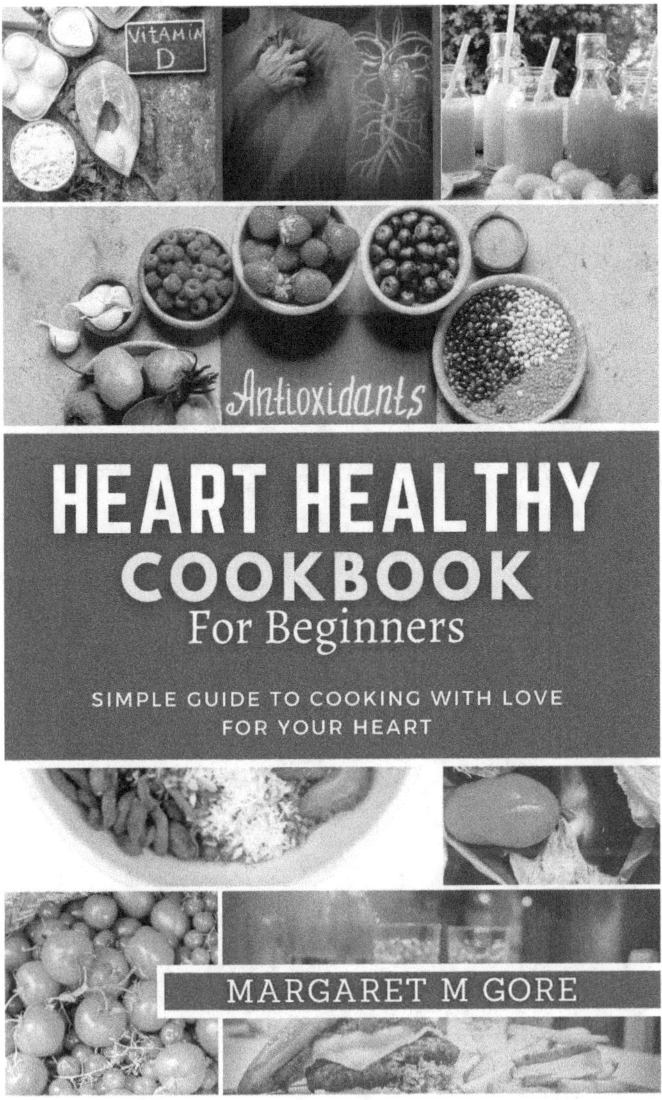

HEART HEALTHY COOKBOOK FOR BEGINNERS

Simple guide to cooking with love for your Heart

Margaret M Gore

damages, or monetary loss due to the information herein, either directly or indirectly.

Respective authors own all copyrights not held by the publisher.

The information herein is offered for informational purposes solely and is universal as so. The presentation of the information is without the contract or any type of guarantee assurance.

The trademarks that are used are without any consent, and the publication of the trademark is without permission or backing by the trademark owner. All trademarks and brands within this book are for clarifying purposes only and are owned by the owners themselves, not affiliated with this document.

Table Of Content

Introduction

The world of heart-healthy cuisine is yours to explore. This cookbook contains a variety of quick, delectable, and healthy dishes that will not only tempt your taste buds but also maintain your heart in top condition. It has never been simpler or more pleasant to eat healthfully.

 You will find straightforward, step-by-step directions for recipes that are bursting with flavor, nutrients, and heart-healthy ingredients, regardless of your level of cooking experience. Let's dive in and explore the wonderful and rewarding world of cooking for your heart.

Considerations For A Heart-healthy Diet

Maintaining a healthy cardiovascular system requires a diet low in saturated fat and cholesterol. This kind of diet lowers the chance of acquiring diabetes, high blood pressure, and stroke in addition to helping to avoid heart disease. Here are 10 compelling arguments for eating a heart-healthy diet.

Lower Cholesterol: A diet high in fiber, produce, whole grains, and cereals help to lower cholesterol levels, which lowers the risk of heart disease.

Reduces Inflammation: Since inflammation is a major contributor to the development of heart disease, a heart-healthy diet low in processed foods and high in antioxidants can help reduce inflammation.

Weight management: A heart-healthy diet can help you maintain a healthy weight, lowering your risk of heart disease and other health issues. This is done by choosing nutrient-dense foods that are low in calories and high in fiber.

Improves Overall Health: Eating a diet high in vitamins, minerals, and vital fatty acids can give the body the resources it needs to perform at its optimum, boosting energy levels.

Increases Heart Health: Foods high in omega-3 fatty acids, such as fish, nuts, and seeds, have been found to increase heart health by lowering blood pressure, reducing inflammation, and boosting blood flow.

Supports Brain Health: Research has shown that eating a diet high in fruits, vegetables, whole grains, and healthy fats will protect against cognitive decline and memory loss as we age.

Reduces Chance of Cancer: Studies have indicated that a diet high in antioxidants, such as fruits and vegetables, can reduce the risk of getting some types of cancer.

Reduces Blood Pressure: It has been demonstrated that a diet high in potassium and low in sodium lowers blood pressure, which lowers the risk of heart disease and stroke.

Reduces the Risk of Digestive Issues: A diet high in fiber and low in processed foods can lower the risk of digestive issues including constipation and irritable bowel syndrome.

Immune System Booster: A heart-healthy diet high in vitamins and minerals can aid in the immune system boosting, lowering the risk of infections, and enhancing general health.

A Description Of Heart Disease And Its Risk Elements

The cardiovascular illness usually referred to as heart disease, is a broad term for several ailments that have an impact on the heart and blood arteries. Coronary artery disease, the most prevalent form of heart disease, is brought on by a buildup of plaque in the arteries that carry blood to the heart muscle. Chest pain, heart attacks, and other severe health issues might result from this.

Heart disease risk factors include:

1. Age: As people get older, their risk of heart disease rises. The danger is larger for people over 65.

2. Gender: Men typically have a higher chance of developing heart disease than women do, while this risk rises for women after menopause.

3. Family history: Your risk is higher if a close relative, such as a parent or brother, has heart disease.

4. Smoking: Smoking increases the risk of developing heart disease. It causes blood vessel damage and raises the chance of blood clots, both of which can result in heart attacks.

5. Hypertension, often known as high blood pressure, is a significant risk factor for heart disease. The heart and blood arteries are subjected to additional strain, and over time, damage may result.

6. High cholesterol: Having high amounts of cholesterol in the blood might make it more likely that the arteries will develop plaque, which can cause heart disease.

7. Diabetes: Diabetics are more likely to develop heart disease, particularly if their

blood sugar levels are not under good control.

8. Being overweight or obese raises your risk of developing heart disease as well as other conditions including high blood pressure and type 2 diabetes.

9. Lack of physical activity: Sedentary behavior raises the risk of heart disease and other conditions like high blood pressure and obesity.

10. Poor diet: A diet heavy in sodium, added sweets, and saturated and trans fats can raise your chance of developing heart disease.

It's crucial to keep in mind that many risk factors can combine to raise your risk of developing heart disease. You can lower your risk and contribute to the prevention of heart disease by leading a healthy lifestyle and cooperating with your doctor.

Knowing The Fundamentals of Heart-healthy Cooking

Making dietary adjustments to reduce the risk of heart disease and other related health problems is the main focus of heart-healthy cooking. The idea is to cook meals that are high in nutrients like fiber, vitamins, and minerals yet low in saturated fat, trans fat, and cholesterol. Here is a detailed guide to learning the fundamentals of heart-healthy cooking.

- **Lessen trans and saturated fats**

Unhealthy fats like trans and saturated fats elevate cholesterol and increase the risk of heart disease. They can be found in processed and fried foods as well as animal products like butter, cheese, and meat. Change to lean meat cuts, choose low-fat dairy products and cut out on processed meals to lower the quantity of saturated and trans fats in your diet.

- **Increased Intake of Fiber**

Because it lowers cholesterol levels and lowers the risk of heart disease, fiber is crucial for a healthy heart. Whole grains, fruits, vegetables, and legumes are good sources of fiber. At least five servings of fruits and vegetables should be included in your diet each day. Whenever possible, choose whole grain items over refined grain products.

- **Use wholesome cooking techniques**

It's crucial to pick healthy cooking techniques while you're cooking that keep the nutrients in your food and cut back on bad fats. Instead of frying your meal, try baking, grilling, or boiling it. Additionally, substitute olive oil for butter or margarine and other unhealthy fats.

- **Reduce Your Sodium Intake**

A key risk factor for heart disease is high blood pressure, which can be brought on by eating too much sodium. Avoid adding salt to your food while it is being prepared or served at the table to lower your sodium intake. Use herbs, spices, and other seasonings to give your food flavor instead. Additionally, select canned and packaged foods that are low in sodium or that are unsalted.

- **Eat heart-healthy foods**

Including heart-healthy items in your diet is essential for lowering your chance of developing heart disease.

The following are some of the top heart-healthy foods:

1. Fatty fish that are high in omega-3 fatty acids, such as salmon, mackerel, and sardines.
2. Seeds and nuts, which are rich sources of fiber and good fats.
3. Berries, which are rich in fiber and antioxidants.
4. dark leafy greens, which are rich in vitamins and minerals and include spinach and kale.

You can protect your heart and lower your risk of heart disease by making these dietary modifications. Always choose healthy options and restrict your intake of bad foods because maintaining a heart-healthy diet is a lifetime commitment.

Chapter 1

Being Aware Of Heart-healthy Eating

Although heart disease is one of the top causes of death in the world, many of its risk factors can be decreased by adopting a balanced diet and other lifestyle adjustments. A heart-healthy diet consists of foods that are high in fiber, vitamins, and minerals and low in saturated and trans fats, cholesterol, sodium, and added sugars.

In this chapter, we will examine the essential elements of a heart-healthy diet, comprehend the relationship between diet and heart health, investigate the many types of fats and their effects on human health, and offer advice and suggestions for selecting heart-healthy foods. You will have a greater awareness of the foods that can support heart health by the end of this article, as well as the measures you can take to develop a heart-healthy eating habits.

The Role Of Nutrients in Heart Healthy Diet

The heart, which is located in the middle of our bodies, is the organ in charge of pumping blood and supplying all of our cells with vital nutrients and oxygen. To avoid heart illnesses, the top cause of mortality worldwide, we must take care of our hearts and maintain a healthy lifestyle. Nutrients are essential for sustaining heart health, and a heart-healthy diet is essential for keeping our hearts in prime condition.

Fiber is one of the most crucial elements of a heart-healthy diet. Foods like oats, barley, and beans include soluble fiber, which lowers cholesterol and lowers the risk of heart disease. Insoluble fiber, which is present in foods like whole grain bread and cereals, on the other hand, encourages regularity and aids in the prevention of constipation.

Another crucial vitamin associated with a lower risk of heart disease is omega-3 fatty acids. These important fatty acids can be obtained through plant-based sources such as flaxseeds, chia seeds, and walnuts as well as fatty fish like salmon, mackerel, and sardines. Blood pressure is lowered, heart health is improved, and inflammation is reduced with the aid of omega-3 fatty acids.

For the maintenance of a healthy heart, potassium is a necessary mineral. By regulating blood pressure, potassium lowers the risk of heart disease and stroke. Bananas, oranges, potatoes, and leafy greens are a few examples of foods high in potassium.

The vitamins B6, B12, and folate are also crucial for keeping the heart healthy. Homocysteine is an amino acid that can damage blood vessels and raise the risk of heart disease. These vitamins aid in regulating homocysteine levels. These vitamins are found in foods including leafy greens, legumes, nuts, and seeds.

A heart-healthy diet must also contain antioxidants, such as vitamins C and E. These vitamins assist in lowering the risk of heart disease and protecting the heart from oxidative stress. Berries, citrus fruits, and leafy greens are examples of foods high in antioxidants.

Sodium is a mineral that is frequently linked to hypertension and a higher risk of heart disease. Sodium intake needs to be decreased if you want to keep your heart healthy. Because packaged and processed meals frequently include a lot of sodium, it's crucial to restrict them and go for natural, unprocessed foods instead.

Finally, a heart-healthy diet should include foods high in mono- and polyunsaturated fats, which may be found in items like olive oil, avocados, and almonds. These heart-healthy fats can aid in reducing inflammation, lowering cholesterol, and strengthening the heart.

Different Types of Fats and How They Affect Heart Health

A balanced diet must include fats since they give our bodies energy and promote general health. But not all fats are made equally. While some forms of fat can be harmful to heart health, others may be advantageous. The most typical fats and their effects on heart health are listed below:

Saturated Fats: Saturated fats can be found in animal products including meat, butter, cheese, and milk. They are normally solid at room temperature. They increase levels of LDL (bad) cholesterol, which can boost the danger of developing heart disease.

Trans Fats: When oils are hydrogenated, a substance is produced that solidifies at room temperature. In processed foods like baked goods, fried foods, and snack foods, they are frequently present. Heart disease risk is increased by trans fats since they have been found to increase LDL cholesterol and decrease HDL (good) cholesterol levels.

Unsaturated fats are present in plant-based oils including olive oil, avocado oil, and nut oils, and are normally liquid at room temperature. By lowering LDL cholesterol levels and raising HDL cholesterol levels, these fats have been found to improve heart health.

Monounsaturated Fats: A form of unsaturated fat, monounsaturated fats can be found in foods including almonds, avocados, and olive oil. They have been demonstrated to improve HDL cholesterol levels and lower LDL cholesterol, which is good for the heart.

Unsaturated fats of the type known as polyunsaturated fats are present in foods like flaxseeds, fatty fish, and walnuts. These fats have been demonstrated to improve HDL cholesterol levels and lower LDL cholesterol, which is good for the heart.

Although unsaturated fats may be good for the heart, it's still vital to eat them in moderation. Even the beneficial unsaturated fats can cause weight gain and other health problems if consumed in excess.

In conclusion, the kind of fat we eat has a big impact on how healthy our hearts are. Unsaturated fats, particularly monounsaturated and polyunsaturated fats, should be ingested in moderation as part of a balanced diet whereas saturated and trans fats should be kept to a minimum. By consuming the right kinds of fats, we can protect our hearts and enhance our general health.

Food Label Comprehension and Heart-healthy Food Selection

Food labels are crucial for assisting us in making educated choices regarding what we eat. But it can be difficult to know what to look for with so much information to process. We are here to assist you in understanding the terminology on food labels so that you can make heart-healthy decisions for yourself and your loved ones.

Saturated and trans fats, salt, and cholesterol are the nutrients to watch out for when it comes to heart health. Consuming foods high in these ingredients raises your risk of heart disease, hypertension, and stroke. It's crucial to choose meals that are high in fiber, vitamins, and minerals while being low in saturated and trans fats, sodium, and cholesterol if you want to reduce your intake of these nutrients.

How do you decide what foods to choose then? The first step is to read the food label. Following are some label components to pay close attention to:

Serving Size: The serving size is the first thing to consider. This is essential since it serves as the foundation for the remaining information on the label. Be sure to compare the serving size to how much you eat. Pay close attention to the serving size.

Total Fat: The amount of fat in a serving is listed in this section. The harmful fats that cause your cholesterol to rise are trans and saturated fats, so pay close attention to the amounts you consume. Choose foods with less than 5% of your daily recommended intake of these fats.

Sodium: It's important to choose foods that are low in sodium because high sodium intake might cause high blood pressure. You should search for foods with less than 140mg of sodium per serving, which is shown on the label for each serving.

Cholesterol: Choosing foods that are low in cholesterol is essential because cholesterol can also contribute to heart disease. Choose foods with less than 20 mg of sodium per serving.

Fiber: Due to its ability to lower cholesterol levels, fiber is crucial for preserving heart health. Be sure to choose foods with at least 3g of fiber per serving.

Nutrients: The vitamins and minerals that are contained in a serving are also listed on the food label. Pick foods with a high concentration of important elements, such as calcium, potassium, and iron, and a few empty calories, such as sugar.

You may make educated judgments and make sure that you're providing your body with the proper nutrients by paying attention to serving sizes, total fat, sodium, cholesterol, fiber, and other nutrients. Therefore, the next time you're shopping, take some time to read the labels and select items that will keep your heart healthy and happy.

Meal Planning and Portion Control

Planning meals and controlling portions are crucial components of cooking for heart health. A balanced diet low in sodium added sweets, and saturated and trans fats can help lower the risk of heart disease and improve general health. Here is detailed instruction on how to organize and manage your meals for a heart-healthy diet.

Meal preparation:

Begin by planning a menu for the following week that features a range of fresh fruits, vegetables, whole grains, lean proteins, and healthy fats.

To keep meals interesting and enticing, use a diversity of colors, flavors, and textures.

To keep track of the food you consume and to assist you in planning and following your diet, use a food diary or meal planning software.

To save time and decrease food waste, make use of leftovers, freezer meals, and batch cooking.

Make healthy replacements, such as switching to whole wheat flour from white flour or fruit and nuts in place of processed treats.

Managing portions:

To precisely measure meals and avoid overeating, use a kitchen scale or measuring cups.

Half of your plate should consist of fruits and vegetables, followed by one-fourth of lean protein and one-fourth of entire grains.

When eating out, especially, stay away from big portion sizes and utilize smaller plates to assist manage quantities.

Eat slowly to give your body time to register that you are full and pay attention to your body's signals of hunger and fullness.

You may maintain a heart-healthy diet, lower your chance of developing heart disease, and improve your general health by incorporating these recommendations into your cooking and eating routines. You can ensure you are getting all the nutrients you need and prevent overeating harmful foods by planning your meals and managing quantities. So get started right away and improve your heart and general wellness!

Maintaining a healthy heart and lowering the risk of cardiovascular disease need heart-friendly nutrition. It's crucial to have a fully equipped kitchen with the appropriate appliances and products to make healthy cooking simpler.

Chapter 2

Heart-healthy Kitchen Essentials

The Basics Of Cooking with Heart healthy oils

There are several advantages to using heart-healthy oils when cooking for our general health and well-being. Certain characteristics of oils that are thought to be heart-healthy include having high concentrations of monounsaturated and polyunsaturated fats and low concentrations of saturated fats. These oils have the potential to lower the risk of heart disease, stroke, and other related illnesses.

The following list includes some of the most popular heart-healthy oils:

One of the most popular oils for heart health is olive oil. It has a lot of monounsaturated fats, which can help lower blood levels of harmful cholesterol and minimize the chance of developing heart disease. Antioxidants found in abundance in olive oil can help guard the body against oxidative damage.

Avocado Oil: Rich in monounsaturated fatty acids, avocado oil is another well-known, heart-healthy oil. Its mild, nutty flavor makes it a fantastic ingredient for a wide range of meals, including salad dressings and stir-fries.

Canola Oil: Canola oil is high in monounsaturated and polyunsaturated fats and low in saturated fats. This makes it a fantastic option for people who want to keep their hearts healthy. Canola oil is useful for cooking because it has a neutral flavor.

Omega-6 and omega-3 fatty acids, as well as polyunsaturated fats, are abundant in sunflower oil. Inflammation, which is a risk factor for heart disease, can be decreased by doing this. Due to its light flavor, sunflower oil is a great option for baking and cooking.

Omega-6 and omega-3 fatty acids are abundant in safflower oil, another oil that is high in polyunsaturated fats. It is a fantastic option for people who want to keep their hearts healthy because it is low in saturated fats. Safflower oil can be utilized in a range of cooking processes and has a mild flavor.

The smoke point of the oil should be taken into account when using heart-healthy oils in cooking. The temperature at which an oil starts to smoke and degrade is referred to as the smoke point. Oils should not be used for cooking if they are heated over their smoke point because doing so might cause them to emit toxic substances and develop bad odors.

Here are some pointers for using heart-healthy oils when cooking:

- Oils should be kept in a cold, dark location to prevent oxidation, which can lower the oil's quality.

- Apply the appropriate oil to the task at hand: Some oils are better suited for high-heat cooking, while others are ideal for drizzling on salads and vegetables.

- Avoid overheating oils because doing so can lead to their breakdown and the release of dangerous substances as well as a reduction in quality.

- Use oils sparingly: Despite the potential health benefits of heart-healthy oils, it's still crucial to use them sparingly. Even so, consuming excessive amounts of oil might harm our health and cause us to gain weight.

It's crucial to use oils that are high in monounsaturated and polyunsaturated fats and low in saturated fats and to use them sparingly when choosing and cooking with them. You can take advantage of the many advantages that heart-healthy oils have to offer by adhering to these recommendations.

PANTRY CONSTRUCTION

Maintaining good heart health requires creating a heart-healthy pantry. A well-stocked pantry is an essential part of a healthy diet and way of life and can aid in the prevention of heart disease and other chronic health issues. We'll go through the necessary steps for creating a heart-healthy pantry in this post, so you can make sure your house is filled with wholesome and delectable foods that promote heart health.

Stock up on heart-healthy essentials as a first step.

Stocking up on staple foods that are high in nutrients and low in harmful fats and added sugars is the first step in creating a pantry that is heart-healthy. Your diet should be based on these foods, which include:

Whole grains: Whole grains have a lot of fiber, which lowers cholesterol and lowers the risk of heart disease. Examples of whole grains are brown rice, quinoa, and whole-wheat bread.

Lentils, chickpeas, and other legumes are excellent sources of fiber and protein. Additionally, they include a lot of vital nutrients including potassium, magnesium, and iron while being low in fat.

Fruits and veggies: Fruits and vegetables are low in calories and high in vitamins, minerals, and antioxidants. To maximize the health advantages, make sure to incorporate a range of vibrant fruits and vegetables into your diet.

Nuts and seeds: Nuts and seeds are a fantastic source of protein, fiber, and good fats. They include a lot of magnesium, potassium, and vitamin E, all of which are heart-healthy vitamins and minerals.

Step 2: Steer clear of packaged and high-fat foods.

To create a pantry that is heart-healthy, avoid processed and high-fat items. These meals frequently include high levels of bad fats, carbohydrates, and salt that can lead to heart disease and other health issues. Don't eat things like:

Fried foods: Fried meals are heavy in unhealthy fats and calories, such as French fries and fried chicken.

Snacks that have been processed: Snacks that have been processed, such as sweets and potato chips, frequently contain a lot of sugar, salt, and bad fats.

High-fat foods: High-fat meats have a lot of saturated and trans fats, which can cause cholesterol levels to rise and increase the risk of heart disease. Examples of high-fat meats are bacon and sausage.

Step 3: Select better options.

It's crucial to select healthier options when buying snacks and other cupboard essentials. Here are some alternatives to think about:

Baked snacks: Baked snacks have less fat and calories than fried snacks, including baked chips and crackers.

Whole-grain crackers: Due to their high fiber content and other nutritional value, whole-grain crackers are a healthier alternative to processed snacks.

Low-fat dairy products are a fantastic source of calcium and other necessary elements. Examples include skim milk and low-fat yogurt.

Olive oil and avocado oil are examples of heart-healthy oils that are preferable to bad fats like butter and lard.

It takes some work to create a heart-healthy pantry, but it's worth it for your long-term well-being. You can create a pantry that supports your heart health and general well-being by stocking up on heart-healthy basics, avoiding processed and high-fat foods, and picking healthier alternatives.

Equipment And Kitchen Tools For Heart-healthy Cooking

Making heart-healthy food might be difficult, especially if you don't know what tools and supplies to use. Here is a list of necessary kitchen appliances and gadgets to make cooking quicker, healthier, and more pleasurable:

Non-Stick Pans: Because they use less oil and can lower the amount of saturated fat in your meals, non-stick pans are a necessity for heart-healthy cooking.

Using a steamer basket, you may prepare vegetables, seafood, and other nutritious meals while preserving their flavor and nutrients.

Salad spinner: To prepare fresh, crisp salads, you'll need one to squeeze out extra water and keep the greens crisp for days.

Measuring cups and spoons are important for proper portion control, which is a vital component of cooking for a healthy heart.

Cutting boards: Invest in a high-quality cutting board to simplify food preparation and lower the possibility of cross-contamination.

A box grater is a multipurpose kitchen appliance that can be used to shred cheese, produce, and fruits for salads and other cuisines.

A useful appliance for mixing sauces, soups, and smoothies is an immersion blender.

Vegetable peeler: To make fruits and vegetables simpler to digest, the skin can be removed with this straightforward but crucial equipment.

A microplane is a tiny grater that can be used to shred cheese, zest citrus fruits, and make garnishes.

Oven thermometer: To ensure that your oven is at the proper temperature, which is necessary for cooking that is good for your heart, you must use an oven thermometer.

You can make cooking heart-healthy meals simpler, better for you, and more pleasurable by investing in some key kitchen gear and supplies. These appliances will enable you to cook scrumptious, nourishing meals that will support the health and happiness of your heart, whether you're just starting or looking to upgrade your kitchen.

How To Understand And Use Spices For Health Benefits And Flavor

Spices are a crucial part of cooking since they provide food taste, scent, and color. However, did you realize that they also provide several health advantages? Knowing how to utilize different spices can improve your cooking and provide more taste and nutrition to your food. In this post, we'll examine the advantages of utilizing spices and how to do so for optimal flavor and health benefits.

Benefits of spices for health
Antioxidants, which shield cells from harm and lessen inflammation, are included in a variety of spices. For instance, turmeric, a key ingredient

in Indian cooking, has anti-inflammatory and powerful antioxidant qualities. Another spice with anti-inflammatory properties that can help with pain relief and swelling is ginger.

Spices have antioxidant effects in addition to helping with digestion, metabolism, and blood sugar control. Black pepper can help boost metabolism and enhance digestion, while cinnamon has been demonstrated to control blood sugar levels and improve insulin sensitivity.

Making use of spices in your cooking
The secret to successfully using spices in cooking is, to begin with, a modest amount and taste as you go. Consider how much you're utilizing because it's simpler to add something than to take something away. To determine which spices you prefer, you can also experiment.

Spices should be used in combination for the best flavor and health advantages. For instance, adding turmeric, ginger, and cinnamon to smoothies, drinks, and baked products can be delectable and healthy.

Using spice rubs is another technique to use spices in your cuisine. Simply combine your preferred spices and spread them onto meats before cooking. You can also season roasted veggies with them.

Preserving spices
It's crucial to store your spices properly if you want to keep them delicious and fresh. Keep them away from heat and moisture in a cool, dark location. To preserve the freshness and protection from the light of your spices, think about investing in sealed containers.

Additionally, labeling your spices can help you keep track of what you have on hand and when it was purchased. Depending on how frequently you use them, it's ideal to change spices every 6 to 12 months because they might lose their strength over time.

In conclusion, applying and comprehending spices can improve your meals and provide several health advantages. Adding spices to your meals is a simple and delectable method to boost flavor and wellness due to their anti-inflammatory effects and improved digestion. Try experimenting with other spices and combinations to experience the additional culinary and health benefits.

Chapter 3

Cardiovascular Recipes

A long and healthy life depends on maintaining good heart health, which is a major public health concern. Eating wholesome, well-balanced meals can help to improve heart health and stave off disease. Each recipe in this book has been thoughtfully created to give the necessary nutrients for a healthy heart. It is delicious and heart-healthy. For those who are busy but still want to eat healthily and take care of their heart health, these recipes are savory, simple to make, and ideal. This book is the ideal tool for you if you want to lower your risk of heart disease, manage current medical conditions, or simply enhance your general health. Prepare your body and palate for nourishment with these delectable, heart-healthy meals!

Breakfast Recipes

Avocado Toast.

Whole grain bread, avocado, salt, pepper, lemon juice, and cherry tomatoes make up an avocado toast.

Toast the toast, then spread it with the avocado mixture and sprinkle it with the cherry tomatoes.

Benefit: Avocados are a wonderful source of fiber and unsaturated fats, which can decrease cholesterol.

Nuts and Berries in Oatmeal

Ingredients: Old-fashioned oats, almond milk, mixed berries, chopped almonds, honey, and cinnamon are the ingredients.

Process: Prepare oats with almond milk, then top with a mixture of berries, chopped nuts, honey, and cinnamon.

Benefit: Oatmeal is a rich source of fiber and berries are high in antioxidants, both of which can assist enhance heart health.

Greek yogurt parfait

Greek yogurt, mixed berries, granola, and honey
are the ingredients for the Greek yogurt parfait.
Procedure: To make, fill a glass with Greek
yogurt, mixed berries, and granola, and drizzle
over the honey.
Benefit: Berries are high in antioxidants, which
can help improve heart health, while Greek
yogurt is a healthy source of calcium and
protein.

Smoothie with peanut butter and banana

Chia seeds, honey, banana, almond milk.
Blend the following ingredients until smooth:
peanut butter, banana, almond milk, chia seeds,
and honey.
Benefit: Bananas are rich in potassium, which
can help lower blood pressure, and peanut butter
is a wonderful source of heart-healthy
unsaturated fats.

Veggie Omelette

Eggs, your choice of vegetables (bell peppers, onions, spinach), cheese, salt, and pepper are the ingredients for the Veggie Omelette.
Beat the eggs, then add the vegetables, cheese, salt, and pepper. Cook until the eggs are set.
Benefit: Vegetables are rich in minerals and fiber and eggs are a wonderful source of protein, both of which can aid to promote heart health.

Breakfast bowl made with sweet potatoes and eggs, with your choice of vegetables (such as bell peppers, onions, spinach), cheese, salt, and pepper.
Process: Scramble eggs, add veggies, cheese, salt, and pepper, then cook chopped sweet potatoes until they are soft. Top with avocado slices when serving.
Benefit: Eggs are a wonderful amount of protein and sweet potatoes are a rich supply of fiber, vitamins, and minerals, all of which can assist enhance heart health.

Yogurt-topped whole-grain waffles with berries

Whole grain waffle mix, mixed berries, Greek yogurt, and honey are the ingredients.

Cook waffles as directed on the package, then top with Greek yogurt, honey, and a mixture of fruit.

Benefit: Mixed berries are rich in antioxidants and whole grain waffles are a wonderful source of fiber, both of which can assist to enhance heart health.

Veggie and Cheese Scramble.

Eggs, your choice of vegetables (bell peppers, onions, spinach), cheese, salt, and pepper are the ingredients for the Veggie and Cheese Scramble. Beat the eggs, then add the vegetables, cheese, salt, and pepper. Cook until the eggs are set.

Benefit: Vegetables are rich in minerals and fiber and eggs are a wonderful source of protein, both of which can aid to promote heart health.

Fruit and Whole Grain Pancakes:

Whole grain pancake mix, mixed fruit, syrup, and butter are the ingredients.

Process: Make pancakes as directed on the package, top with syrup and mixed fruit, then plate with a dollop of butter.

Benefit: Mixed fruit is rich in vitamins and minerals and whole grain pancakes are a wonderful source of fiber, both of which can support heart health.

Recipes For Appetizers And Snacks

Sweet Potato Fries Baked

2 medium sweet potatoes, peeled and chopped into thin sticks, are the ingredients.

Olive oil, 1 tbsp

To taste, add salt and pepper.

Process:

Set the oven to 425 °F.

Use parchment paper to cover a baking sheet.

Slices of sweet potato should be mixed with olive oil, salt, and pepper in a big bowl.

Slices of sweet potato should be arranged on the baking sheet in a single layer.

Cook for 20 to 25 minutes, or until golden and crispy.

Benefit: Sweet potatoes are a heart-healthy snack option because they are a wonderful source of fiber and antioxidants. Another way to reduce harmful fat is to bake rather than fry.

Roasted chickpeas

Ingredients for roasted chickpeas: 1 can be rinsed and drained chickpeas.
Olive oil, 1 tbsp
spices, and salt of your choosing (such as paprika or cumin)
Process:Set the oven to 400 °F.
Use parchment paper to cover a baking sheet.
Chickpeas should be combined with olive oil, salt, and spices in a big bowl.
On the prepared baking sheet, spread the chickpeas out in a single layer.
Cook for 20 to 25 minutes, or until golden and crispy.
Benefit: Chickpeas are a heart-healthy snack option since they are a wonderful source of fiber and plant-based protein. The chickpeas gain a nice crunch from roasting without getting any extra fat.

Hummus and Veggie Sticks

Ingredients: Various raw veggies, including bell peppers, carrots, celery, and cucumbers
1 hummus cup
Process: Vegetables should be washed and sliced into thin sticks.Serve a side of hummus on the side for dipping the veggie sticks.
Benefit: Consuming a variety of raw veggies is an excellent method to obtain essential vitamins and minerals, and hummus is a heart-healthy dip alternative prepared from fiber-rich chickpeas and heart-healthy olive oil.

Edamame

1 cup shelled edamame Salt to taste
Process: Water should be heated up in a pot. When the water is boiling, add the edamame and cook for 3 to 5 minutes, or until soft.
If desired, drain and sprinkle salt.
Benefit: Edamame is a heart-healthy snack option because it's a wonderful source of fiber and plant-based protein.

Baked Sweet Potato Fries.

4 medium sweet potatoes, 2 tbsp olive oil, 1 tsp paprika, 1 tsp garlic powder, salt, and pepper are the ingredients for baked sweet potato fries.
The oven should be heated to 400 degrees. Sweet potatoes should be thinly sliced. Add oil, paprika, garlic powder, salt, and pepper to the mixture. 20 to 25 minutes of baking.
Benefit: Sweet potatoes are an excellent source of fiber, antioxidants, vitamins, and minerals.

Veggie Sticks With Hummus Dip

Carrots, cucumbers, bell peppers, cherry tomatoes, and hummus are the ingredients for veggie sticks with hummus dip.
Cut vegetables into sticks as a process. Serve hummus on the side for dipping.
Benefit: Vegetables lessen the risk of heart disease since they are high in fiber, vitamins, and minerals while being low in calories.

Grilled Eggplant

1 large eggplant, 2 tablespoons of olive oil, salt, pepper, lemon juice, and basil are the ingredients for grilled eggplant.
Slice the eggplant into rounds to prepare. Apply oil to the surface and season with basil, lemon juice, salt, and pepper. Grill each side for two to three minutes.
Benefit: Rich in fiber, vitamins, and minerals, eggplant is a low-calorie, low-fat, and low-carb vegetable.

Spinach And Feta Stuffed Tomatoes

Four large tomatoes, one cup of spinach, half a cup of feta cheese, a quarter cup of breadcrumbs, and one clove of garlic, salt, pepper, and olive oil make up the spinach and feta stuffed tomatoes recipe.
Cut each tomato's top off, then remove the seeds with a spoon. Combine the breadcrumbs, spinach, feta, garlic, salt, and pepper. After stuffing each tomato with the mixture, add little oil. At 375°F, bake for 20 minutes.

Benefit: Spinach is a good source of antioxidants, vitamins, and minerals, all of which support heart health.

Salad Of Grilled Peaches And Burrata

The salad of grilled peaches and burrata contains the following ingredients: arugula, balsamic sauce, olive oil, salt, and pepper.

Procedure: Halve the peaches, then remove the pit. Grill each side for three to four minutes. Burrata cheese should be served with arugula and a balsamic sauce, as well as oil, salt, and pepper.

Benefit: Peaches are a fruit low in calories but high in fiber, vitamins, and minerals that help reduce the risk of heart disease.

Stuffed Bell Peppers.

4 bell peppers, 1 cup cooked quinoa, 1 can black beans, 1 cup corn, 1 diced tomato, 1 diced onion, 1 clove garlic, 1 tsp cumin, salt, pepper, and

cilantro are the ingredients for stuffed bell peppers.

Process: Turn the oven on to 375°F. Bell peppers should have their tops cut off and their seeds are taken out. Quinoa, black beans, corn, tomato, onion, garlic, cumin, salt, pepper, and cilantro should all be combined in a bowl. After baking for 30 minutes, fill each pepper with the mixture.

Benefit: Bell peppers are a high-fiber, low-calorie veggie.

Entrees

Salmon with Herbs on the Grill:

4 salmon filets, 2 tbsp olive oil, 2 tsp dried basil,
2 tsp dried thyme, salt, pepper, and lemon are the
ingredients.

Process: Combine olive oil, basil, thyme, salt,
and pepper in a bowl. Grill the salmon fillets for
4-5 minutes on each side, or until fully done,
after brushing with the marinade. Serve with a
lemon squeeze.

Benefits: Omega-3 fatty acids, which are
abundant in salmon, can help reduce the risk of
heart disease.

Lentil and Vegetable Stew

One cup of green lentils, two carrots, two celery
stalks, one onion, two garlic cloves, one can of
diced tomatoes, four cups of vegetable broth,
two tablespoons of olive oil, salt, and pepper
make up the Lentil and Vegetable Stew.

The onion, garlic, carrots, and celery should be sautéed in olive oil in a large pot until tender. Lentils, tomatoes, broth, salt, and pepper should be added. When the lentils are ready, simmer them for 25 to 30 minutes after bringing them to a boil.

Benefits: Vegetables include important vitamins and minerals, and lentils are a fantastic source of fiber and protein.

Tacos with baked sweet potatoes and black beans

8 whole wheat tortillas, 4 medium sweet potatoes, 1 can of black beans, 1 teaspoon each of chili powder, cumin, paprika, garlic powder, salt, and pepper (such as avocado, salsa, and cilantro).

The oven should be heated to 400 degrees. The sweet potatoes should be peeled, cut into 1-inch pieces, and placed on a baking pan. Add the seasonings, then bake for 25 to 30 minutes, or until the vegetables are soft. The black beans should be warmed up in a pan. Add chosen toppings after stuffing each tortilla with the sweet potato and black bean mixture.

Benefits: Black beans are a fantastic source of protein and fiber, and sweet potatoes are high in antioxidants.

Grilled Chicken Salad With Quinoa

Ingredients for grilled chicken salad with quinoa include 4 skinless, boneless chicken breasts, 1 cup quinoa, 2 cups water, 2 tablespoons each of olive oil and balsamic vinegar, salt, and pepper, as well as your choice of greens (such as spinach or arugula) and garnishes (such as cherry tomatoes, cucumber, and avocado).

Process: Heat the quinoa and water to a boil in a medium saucepan. Reduce heat, cover, and simmer for 18 to 20 minutes, or until thoroughly done. Combine the olive oil and balsamic vinegar in a basin. Grill the chicken for 5-7 minutes on each side, or until fully cooked, after brushing it with the marinade. Serve the chicken over a bed of greens with your choice of quinoa, veggies, and garnishes.

Benefits: Whole chicken provides lean protein, quinoa is a complete protein and strong in fiber, and greens are a powerhouse of vitamins and minerals.

Salmon On The Grill With Avocado Salsa

Contains four salmon filets.
ripe avocado, with salt and pepper to taste
half a red onion
1 lime, juiced, and 1 tiny jalapeño pepper
1 tablespoon of olive oil
uncooked cilantro
Process: Set the grill's temperature to medium-high.
Add salt and pepper to the salmon to season it.
Combine the diced avocado, red onion, seeded and minced jalapeno, cilantro, lime juice, and olive oil in a small bowl.
Grill the salmon for four to five minutes on each side, or until it is well done.
Serve fish with salsa made from avocados.

Benefits: Omega-3 fatty acids, which are good for the heart and can lower inflammation, are abundant in salmon. Monounsaturated fats, which are abundant in avocado and are good for the heart, are also advantageous.

Quinoa and Vegetable Stir-Fry

Ingredients:
1 cup quinoa
1 tbsp olive oil
1 onion, chopped
3 garlic cloves, minced
1 red bell pepper, sliced
1 yellow squash, sliced
1 cup cherry tomatoes
Salt and pepper to taste
Process: Cook quinoa according to package instructions.
In a large wok or skillet, heat olive oil over medium-high heat.
Add onion and garlic, cook for 2-3 minutes or until fragrant.

Add sliced red bell pepper, yellow squash, and cherry tomatoes. Cook for an additional 4-5 minutes or until vegetables are tender.

Stir in cooked quinoa and season with salt and pepper to taste.

Benefits: Quinoa is a nutrient-rich grain that is high in protein and fiber, making it a great option for heart-healthy cooking. The vegetables in this stir-fry provide important vitamins and minerals and are low in saturated fat.

Lentil and Kale Soup

Ingredients:

1 tbsp olive oil

1 onion, chopped

3 garlic cloves, minced

1 cup green lentils

6 cups vegetable broth

1 large bunch of kale, chopped

Salt and pepper to taste

Process: In a large pot, heat olive oil over medium heat.

Add onion and garlic, cook for 2-3 minutes or until fragrant.
Stir in green lentils, vegetable broth, and chopped kale.
Bring to a boil, then reduce heat and simmer for 20-25 minutes or until lentils are tender.
Season with salt and pepper to taste.
Benefits: Lentils are a great source of fiber and protein, and have been shown to have heart-healthy benefits. Kale is high in antioxidants and other nutrients that can help reduce inflammation and promote heart health.

Side Dishes

Grilled Vegetables:

Ingredients: Bell peppers, zucchini, onions, cherry tomatoes, olive oil, salt, and pepper.
Process: Cut vegetables into similar sizes, brush with olive oil, sprinkle with salt and pepper, and grill on high heat for 10-15 minutes or until tender.
Benefit: Low in fat and calories, high in fiber and vitamins.

Quinoa Salad:

Ingredients: Quinoa, cherry tomatoes, cucumber, red onion, lemon juice, olive oil, salt, and pepper.
Process: Cook quinoa according to instructions, let cool, mix with chopped vegetables, lemon juice, olive oil, salt, and pepper.
Benefit: Rich in protein, fiber, and antioxidants.

Baked Sweet Potato Fries

Ingredients: Sweet potatoes, olive oil, salt, and pepper.

Process: Cut sweet potatoes into thin strips, brush with olive oil, sprinkle with salt and pepper, and bake in the oven at 400°F for 20-25 minutes.

Benefit: Low in fat, high in fiber, and rich in vitamins and antioxidants.

Roasted Brussels Sprouts

Ingredients: Brussels sprouts, olive oil, salt, and pepper.

Process: Cut off the ends of the Brussels sprouts, toss with olive oil, salt, and pepper, and roast in the oven at 400°F for 20-25 minutes or until tender.

Benefit: Low in fat and calories, high in fiber and vitamins.

Broccoli and Cauliflower Stir-Fry

Ingredients: Broccoli, cauliflower, olive oil, garlic, salt, and pepper.
Process: Cut broccoli and cauliflower into bite-sized pieces, heat olive oil in a pan, add garlic, broccoli, and cauliflower, stir-fry for 5-7 minutes or until tender, sprinkle with salt and pepper.
Benefit: Low in fat and calories, high in fiber, vitamins, and antioxidants.

Brown Rice Pilaf:

Ingredients: Brown rice, onion, garlic, vegetable broth, salt, and pepper.
Process: Cook rice according to instructions, in a pan sauté onion and garlic until tender, add vegetable broth and rice, simmer for 10-15 minutes, season with salt and pepper.
Benefit: Rich in fiber, vitamins, and minerals, low in fat and calories.

Desserts Recipe

Baked Apples

Ingredients: 4 medium apples, 2 tbsp. brown sugar, 1 tsp. cinnamon, 1 tsp. vanilla extract, 1/4 cup water

Process: Preheat the oven to 375°F. Core the apples and place them in a baking dish. Mix the brown sugar, cinnamon, and vanilla extract in a small bowl and fill the centers of the apples with the mixture. Pour the water into the dish, cover with foil, and bake for 25-30 minutes or until the apples are tender.

Benefits: Apples are a great source of fiber, which can help lower cholesterol levels.

Banana Oat Cookies

Ingredients: 2 ripe bananas, 1 cup rolled oats, 1/4 cup almond flour, 1 tsp. baking powder, 1 tsp. vanilla extract

Process: Preheat the oven to 350°F. Mash the bananas in a bowl and mix in the oats, almond

flour, baking powder, and vanilla extract. Drop spoonfuls of the mixture onto a baking sheet lined with parchment paper and bake for 12-15 minutes or until the edges are golden brown.
Benefits: Oats are high in soluble fiber, which helps lower cholesterol levels. Almond flour is a good source of healthy unsaturated fats.

Chia Seed Pudding

Ingredients: 1 cup almond milk, 2 tbsp. chia seeds, 1 tsp. vanilla extract, 1 tbsp. honey
Process: Mix the almond milk, chia seeds, vanilla extract, and honey in a bowl. Let the mixture sit in the fridge for at least 30 minutes or until it thickens into a pudding-like consistency.
Benefits: Chia seeds are high in fiber, omega-3 fatty acids, and antioxidants, all of which are beneficial for heart health.

Frozen Yogurt Bark

Ingredients: 2 cups Greek yogurt, 1/4 cup honey, 1 tsp. vanilla extract, 1 cup mixed berries

Process: Mix the yogurt, honey, and vanilla extract in a bowl. Pour the mixture onto a parchment-lined baking sheet and spread it out evenly. Top with the mixed berries and freeze for at least 2 hours or until firm. Break the bark into pieces and serve.

Benefits: Greek yogurt is a good source of protein and probiotics, which can improve heart health. Berries are high in antioxidants and fiber.

Grilled Peaches

Ingredients: 4 ripe peaches, 1 tsp. cinnamon, 1 tsp. vanilla extract, 1 tbsp. honey

Process: Preheat a grill to medium heat. Cut the peaches in half and remove the pits. Mix the cinnamon, vanilla extract, and honey in a small bowl and brush the mixture onto the cut sides of the peaches. Place the peaches on the grill, cut side down, and cook for 3-4 minutes or until grill marks appear.

Benefits: Peaches are a good source of fiber and vitamins, which are important for heart health.

Strawberry Sorbet

Ingredients: 2 cups strawberries, 1/2 cup sugar, 1/2 cup water, 1 tsp. lemon juice

Process: Blend the strawberries in a food processor until smooth. In a small saucepan, heat the sugar and water over medium heat until the sugar dissolves. Mix the sugar syrup with the blended strawberries and lemon juice in a blender. Pour the mixture into a container and freeze for at least 4 hours or until firm. Scoop and serve.

Benefits: Strawberries are high in antioxidants and vitamin C,

Chapter 4

Heart-Healthy Meal Planning and Prep

Eating a healthy and balanced diet is important for maintaining good health and reducing the risk of heart disease. A heart-healthy diet should include a variety of nutrient-dense foods, such as fruits, vegetables, whole grains, lean proteins, and healthy fats.

Meal Planning Tips And Tricks

Heart healthy cooking and meal planning are essential for maintaining good cardiovascular health. Here are some tips and tricks to help beginners get started:

Know your dietary needs: Understanding your dietary needs, such as the recommended daily intake of nutrients and the types of food that you should limit or avoid, is the first step to heart-healthy cooking and meal planning.

Plan your meals in advance: Planning your meals in advance helps you stick to healthy food choices and prevents last-minute junk food cravings. Try to plan your meals for the week and make a grocery list to ensure that you have all the ingredients you need.

Focus on whole, unprocessed foods: Incorporating whole, unprocessed foods into your meals, such as fruits, vegetables, lean proteins, and whole grains, can help lower your risk of heart disease. Try to limit your intake of processed foods, which are often high in unhealthy fats, salt, and sugar.

Use heart-healthy cooking methods: When cooking, try to use healthy cooking methods such as grilling, baking, or roasting, instead of deep-frying or sautéing in large amounts of oil.

Control portion sizes: Consuming smaller portions can help you control your calorie intake and maintain a healthy weight, which is essential for good heart health.

Watch your salt intake: High salt intake can increase your blood pressure, which is a risk factor for heart disease. Try to limit your salt intake by avoiding processed foods and adding salt sparingly when cooking.

Use healthy fats: Incorporating healthy fats, such as olive oil, avocado, and nuts, into your meals can help lower your risk of heart disease. Try to limit your intake of unhealthy fats, such as saturated and trans fats, which are found in processed foods and fatty meats.

Incorporate physical activity: Physical activity is essential for maintaining good heart health. Try to incorporate physical activity into your daily routine, such as taking a walk or going to the gym.

How To Make Healthy Meals In Advance

Making healthy meals in advance is a great way to save time and ensure that you have nutritious options available throughout the week. Here's how to get started:

Plan your meals: Decide on the meals you want to make for the week and create a grocery list based on the ingredients you need.

Shop for ingredients: Stock up on fresh fruits, vegetables, lean proteins, and whole grains, as well as pantry staples such as spices, olive oil, and vinegar.

Prep your ingredients: Wash and chop your fruits and vegetables, and cook and store your proteins. For example, you could bake chicken breasts, cook a pot of brown rice, or steam some broccoli.

Assemble your meals: Use containers to portion out your ingredients into individual meals. You could make salads, wraps, or grain bowls, or simply store ingredients separately so you can mix and match as needed.

Store in the refrigerator: Keep your pre-made meals in the refrigerator or freezer until you're ready to eat them.

Reheat and enjoy: When you're ready for a meal, simply reheat in the microwave or on the stove and enjoy a nutritious, home-cooked meal that you prepared in advance.

Remember to keep food safety in mind, always refrigerate perishable items and be mindful of the shelf life of your meals.

Tips For Eating Out While Maintaining A Heart-healthy Diet

Here are some tips for eating out while maintaining a heart-healthy diet:

Look for menu items that are grilled, baked, broiled, or steamed, rather than fried.
Choose dishes that are rich in fiber, such as vegetables, whole grains, and legumes.
Opt for lean proteins, such as grilled chicken, fish, or tofu.
Ask for dressings, sauces, and condiments on the side so you can control the amount you use.
Avoid menu items that are high in saturated and trans fats, salt, and added sugars.
Ask for nutrition information or special requests, such as modifying menu items to reduce salt and fat content.
Share a meal or take half of it to-go to reduce portion sizes.

Drink water or unsweetened beverages, rather than sugary drinks.

By following these tips, you can make healthier choices when eating out and maintain a heart-healthy diet. It's important to remember that small changes can make a big impact on your overall health.

Conclusion

The Importance Of A Consistent, Heart-healthy Lifestyle

A consistent, heart-healthy lifestyle is essential to maintaining a healthy heart and preventing heart disease. Heart disease is the leading cause of death in the world, but it is largely preventable through lifestyle choices and habits. A heart-healthy lifestyle includes maintaining a healthy diet, being physically active, avoiding tobacco, and managing stress and anxiety.

Eating a balanced and nutritious diet is crucial for a healthy heart. This includes consuming plenty of fruits, vegetables, whole grains, lean proteins, and healthy fats, while limiting the intake of saturated and trans fats, salt, and added sugars. A diet that is high in fiber, potassium, and antioxidants is especially beneficial for heart health.

Physical activity is another important aspect of a heart-healthy lifestyle. Regular exercise can help lower blood pressure, maintain a healthy weight, and reduce the risk of heart disease. Aim to get at least 30 minutes of moderate-intensity physical activity most days of the week. This can include activities such as brisk walking, cycling, swimming, or playing sports.

Tobacco use is a major risk factor for heart disease and should be avoided. Smoking and using tobacco products can damage the heart and blood vessels, leading to serious health problems, including heart attack, stroke, and high blood pressure. If you use tobacco, quitting is the best thing you can do for your heart and overall health.

Finally, managing stress and anxiety is essential for a healthy heart. Stress can lead to high blood pressure and increase the risk of heart disease. It is important to find healthy ways to manage stress, such as practicing relaxation techniques, exercising, or spending time with friends and family.

In conclusion, a consistent, heart-healthy lifestyle is essential for maintaining a healthy heart and preventing heart disease. This includes eating a balanced and nutritious diet, being physically active, avoiding tobacco, and managing stress and anxiety. By making these simple lifestyle choices, you can protect your heart and improve your overall health.

Final Thoughts And Encouragement On Heart-healthy Cooking For Beginners

As a professional in the field of nutrition, I strongly encourage everyone to embrace heart-healthy cooking. Here are a few tips for beginners:

Focus on whole, unprocessed foods: Fruits, vegetables, whole grains, lean proteins, and healthy fats are all key components of a heart-healthy diet.

Limit saturated and trans fats: These types of fats can raise cholesterol levels and increase the risk of heart disease. Opt for unsaturated fats, such as those found in nuts, seeds, and avocados.

Use healthy cooking methods: Bake, broil, grill, or steam your foods instead of frying. This helps to reduce the amount of unhealthy fats and oils that can contribute to heart disease.

Watch portion sizes: Eating too much of any type of food, even healthy foods, can lead to weight gain and increase the risk of heart disease. Pay attention to portion sizes and use a food scale if needed.

Experiment with spices and herbs: Add flavor to your dishes without adding unhealthy fats or salt by using herbs and spices.

Cooking for your heart health can be a fun and delicious experience. Start small, try new recipes, and don't be afraid to experiment. With a little effort and creativity, you can create heart-healthy meals that you and your family will love.